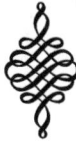

How To Seduce A Woman Without Even Talking To Her

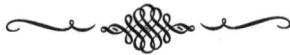

Understanding Women

By

Fritz Gerald Morissette

COPYRIGHT

All rights reserved.

Table of Contents

❧

INTRODUCTION

Are you able to work your magic on any woman and charm her to the point of seduction? You might not believe that you can, but you can learn the guaranteed techniques to charm any woman. You will even learn how to do it with her even knowing it is happening.

I do not care what you think; you cannot seduce a woman by talking to her. She will be listening to what you are saying, but she will be looking for any reason to reject you.

You will get different answers if you ask experts how to seduce a woman. Some of them will tell you not to do anything and leave situations to evolve as you go along. If something is going to happen between you two, it will happen on its own, and there is no dearth of experts who will tell you that to seduce a woman, you need to be prepared for a psychological game and make the right moves.

Seduction is the art of distracting a woman away from all of your shortcomings to find out who you really are. The most seductive way of letting a woman find out who you are is by allowing her to find out on her own rather than talking about yourself a lot.

Important! When you find a woman to talk to, and the conversation is going well, you have to really keep your mind on the "process" to seduce a woman. Remember, this is not about rushing. You want to take things step by step; you may even have to back up and start over from a different angle when trying to seduce a woman. No two women are exactly the same. A great conversation is "hey guys," and using the right words at the most valuable time to seduce a woman.

CHAPTER ONE

❦

UNDERSTANDING WHAT A WOMAN WANTS!

The great question that many men have not been able to answer is "what does a woman want?" Women appear to be a mystery to many men, holding secrets deep inside their hearts. Husbands are often found complaining about their inability to understand their wives even after years of marriage. So what is the reality behind this mystery that's become an obstacle in a relationship?

There are dominant women, there women who are very demanding, and there are wives who nag and impose their decisions on their husbands, but these are just a few exceptions on which a million jokes are created and circulated to mock at womanhood and satisfy the ego of men, who create an impression that women are the root cause of all the difficulties in a relationship. Women, in general, are not very expressive about their feelings, they are brought up in such a way that they always think for and care about others more than themselves.

Change is the constant factor in a woman's life and post marriage a woman has to adjust to new people and adapt to new surroundings. A woman often gives up everything, her home, her parents, her comfort zone, her lifestyle, and her priorities to be with her husband. Men have it easy in this case as there is hardly any difference to life post marriage. In the process of adjustment to an entirely new world for the sake of love, there is hardly any room for personal desires. According to society, this is the norm every woman is born to conform to, yet it's easier said than done.

During courtship men go to any lengths to woo their lady—love, pamper them and give them a lot of attention. Once married, men take their wives for granted and need special occasions to express their love for their lady. As the years go by, men even forget their anniversaries and wife's birthday. When women get upset about these things, men think it is too trivial to be given a thought. Women are very emotional by nature and they invest a lot of effort into remembering details about personal life, such as birthdays, anniversaries or the first date!

Women look for honesty in a man; they often have their insecurities about a man's attitude due to past relationships.

The other trait women look for in a man is Intelligence. Very few women want to go out with men who are not intelligent. Most want to be with a man that others would be awestruck by. They want someone who can show off his college degrees or honor rolls. The third important factor is a guy's financial standing. No woman wants to date a guy who is financially broke until and unless she is really in love.

A woman will be loyal to a man if he goes through a financial crisis after they have been in a relationship, but to start with she would want some sort of financial maturity to exist. Women appreciate a sense of humor; they want their guy to make others laugh, a shy guy is not every girl's dream. They want their guy to make their parents, friends—everyone laugh. The other thing that women look for in a man is his etiquette.

No woman wants to date a guy who right on the first date tells her to pay. Women want their guys to treat them nicely and to follow the proper decorum. It is necessary for them to feel confident they can take their partner out with other friends and not feel embarrassed. Women also want to be physically attracted to a guy, so sensual cologne wouldn't be a bad idea, as well as a guy's attire also matters and so does the model of his car.

Unconditional love, care, understanding, respect, trust, and honesty; these are just a few things, but there is a lot more to what a woman wants. It is the mystery surrounding women that keep men constantly going crazy about them. So take some time off and rediscover your love for your lady!

CHAPTER TWO

HOW TO HAVE POWER AND CONFIDENCE WITH WOMEN

There's nothing scarier for a guy who is interested in a girl than to hear her say, "no." Just consider it. This tiny little word has transformed countless men into nervous wrecks. No one's going to deny that getting shot down is hard to endure, but you've got to keep perspective. If you really want to be successful but can't gain any ground, then now may be the time to change up your game—before all the good women are gone.

MISTAKES TO AVOID AROUND WOMEN

Mistake #1: Not Getting Out of the House (Or Apt.)

Approach women now! Women aren't going to come to you. The absolute best way to start learning how to gain confidence with women is by simply putting yourself out in public and working on your social skills. Talk to everyone, not just girls, and just be a social guy. The more you do this, the easier it will become over time. Before you know it, you'll start finding yourself in the type of situations you now feel you're lacking. Being out multiple times per week also just simply increases your chances of good things happening for you. There are too many guys out there (and I used to be one of them, for a long time) that would gain confidence with women faster if they just simply went out more. I know this sounds like common sense, but trust me, everything changed for me the day I realized I didn't need to read or study one more book, or listen to or watch one more seminar.

Don't be the guy that has to know everything about how to meet beautiful women before he does anything. You're never going to know everything before you even start. Practicing what you're learning by going out and applying it at the same time, supplements what you have learned and helps you understand it all better.

Mistake #2: Worrying Too Much About What A Woman Is Thinking About Them

Guys, it's such an enormous mistake to fall into the trap of getting caught up in your own head. These will circumvent your success in so many ways. Here's a very ironic discovery that I made a couple of years ago: I get more bad reactions from women when, in my head, I'm thinking too long about what I should say before I say it. This is very important so I want you to mull this over for a minute.

When I go through the quick process (2-3 seconds) of going into my head and thinking about "just the right thing to say," it usually gets a bad response, from women and men actually. Why is this? Its because they can sense that you are coming from a place of neediness, i.e. it was important that what you said be positively accepted. What's ironic of course is that "needing something to work out" usually drives it away from you.

In a social environment, no one ever wants to feel awkward or be in the presence of someone who is coming from a place of neediness (as subtle as it may be in this example). It makes people uncomfortable. On the other hand, this is a much better place to come from:

"I trust that most of the time, I have great things to say, so I'll just respond, naturally and without overthinking, and if what I say isn't received well, then oh well, because I know most of the time it is."

This frame subconsciously makes everyone feel more relaxed around you. You aren't "needing" anything. Think about it, when you're out to dinner with someone, and their food is taking too long, you start to feel more uncomfortable the more needy they get about their order. It is no different when a woman is talking to a man that "needs" whatever he says to be funny, it's just on a smaller more unconscious scale. Don't worry about what she thinks! If you're a great guy, chances are very high (if she's a great girl), she'll recognize that.

Mistake #3: Making Rejection Real

Let me give you a secret I learned about how to gain confidence with women: Rejection is only a concept that you made up in your head. A belief is a thought that you make real. As you've grown up, society has presented you with this thought that it's possible to get rejected, one way or another. You took this thought and made it real by turning it into a BELIEF.

You started to believe, at an early age, without questioning it, that yes I can get rejected and yes I need to avoid rejection at all costs. This same process happened when you formed the thought that you have "no confidence with women." You made this real as well by turning the thought into a belief.

Rejection is not real because if you think about it, what have you lost? You didn't have her interest before you approached, and you don't have it now. You didn't lose anything! "But Ash, it's not about protecting what I already have it's about getting something I don't have yet." And my answer to that would be: There's that neediness again, why, why, why do you need her approval? Why can't you just be social and put yourself out there and if she's receptive, then great, wonderful. When you come from a place of non-neediness, its impossible to get rejected. Let me say that again:

When you come from a place of non-neediness, it's not possible to get rejected!

Mistake #4: Believing That Confidence Is Something All Guys Who Are Successful With Women Were Just Born With

While it is true that everyone has different personalities and some guys were just lucky enough to be born into natural self-confidence with women, that certainly doesn't mean you can develop these traits within yourself. Gaining confidence with women is a skill that you can learn, and then become. Take being good at playing a musical instrument for example, like guitar. Everyone who is excellent at guitar had to learn how to play at one point or another. Building confidence within yourself is a skillset you can learn and hone over time. My best advice is to get out there and start talking with people as often as possible. The quicker you learn how to be social with people, the faster you'll become confident in how you relate to other people. This is especially true with women. Other things you can do to gain confidence with women include: Getting into great physical shape, reciting daily affirmations out loud to yourself, and using visual exercises through NLP (Neuro-Linguistic Programming).

Mistake #5: Not Taking Advantage Of The Power Of Body Language and Non-Verbal Communication

It's often the simplest things that make the biggest difference. Studies have shown that 80-90% of what we communicate to other people is unspoken. In other words, non-verbal communication. It would benefit you to such a large degree if you would take the time to study body language. You can sub-communicate so many things at once through body language and that's why it's so powerful. Do you agree that you can tell a lot about a person from the way they dress? Of course, what you gather is not set in stone, but most of the time it's usually pretty accurate. Body language is the same way. The best body language tips I can give you include:

- Making and holding eye contact
- Making slower movements
- Being less reactive to other people than they are to you
- Standing and walking straight with shoulders held slightly back
- Smiling
- Not leaning in while talking to her
- Voice tonality and pace (e.g., not speaking too quickly, adding pauses). This has nothing to do with verbal content or what's being said.

Mistake #6: Getting Her Phone Number With No Specific Intent

There was time when I thought (as I'm sure many inexperienced guys do) that once I got her number, that was it, I had her. This couldn't be further from the truth. A phone number is useless unless you have a specific reason for getting it. A sub-mistake related to this that I see guys do is they'll ask for the number prematurely as well. In fact, she's so used to guys doing this that she's probably desensitized to it and by the time you talk to her, she has been socially programmed to just give her number out, like she did to the 10 guys before you.

To be frank, you'd really have to be bad to not be able to get her number after 5 minutes of talking to her, in most cases anyway. Single, attractive women give their numbers out all the time, the difference lies in how you ask for it.

Think of it from the frame of: "I'm gonna give this girl a chance to get to know me, if I decide she'd be cool to spend time with, I'll set up a meet up with her, and get her number while I'm coordinating that with her." Unless pressed for time, I'd really advise talking to her anywhere between 7-12 minutes, at least, and getting to know her a little, before setting up a meet up/getting her number. Think of it like, she passed your "cool/not cool test," and her prize is that you're going to ask for her number (while making plans). Coming from this frame will also help you in building confidence with women in general, with time and practice.

Mistake #7: Not Approaching Or Opening When The Opportunity Arises

So you've gotten yourself out of the house? Great! But you now need to know how to meet beautiful women when you're out. Going out and just standing around with a beer held to your chest is not going to get you anywhere. Women are not going to approach you. If you're a good-looking guy and you're dressed well, this will happen sometimes, but it's ultimately your job as the man to take the initiative and talk to them. You've got to stop constantly worrying about what could go wrong by going over and opening her. Realize and accept the fact that it's very possible you will catch her in a bad mood or at a bad time, and that's OK.

More often than not, if you approach with a smile, good body language, and strong voice tonality, she'll be more than happy to talk to you. Women go out expecting to get approached, especially attractive women, they're used to having men looking to meet them, it's no big deal. In other words, it's not like you're doing anything out there or unorthodox by approaching her. Try to calibrate yourself to the situation of course, and approaching her from behind is not a good idea, but what's important is that you have the mentality: Approach Women Now.

Mistake #8: Not Using Humor Enough (Or Any), While Interacting With Her

I cannot stress enough the importance of using humor when learning to gain confidence with women. Don't take this to mean you should go into your head (always a huge mistake) and start rapidly thinking of jokes or one-liners to say. What I mean here is just going out with a natural, easygoing vibe and grabbing opportunities to be witty as they present themselves. A girl will usually give you many opportunities to bust her balls and tease her during an interaction. Once you do this a few times, you'll naturally start to get better at it and be able to spot these opportunities.

Women LOVE a man that can do this, they love a man that isn't afraid to tease/poke fun at her a little and can take it from her as well. Its shows you are socially intelligent and that you "get it." It shows you have self-confidence with women. It also makes the interaction fun and more relaxed. Also remember that much like conversation, humor is not linear, meaning if you tease her about something, you can loop back to it again at a later point and tease her again about it. This creates a sense that both of you have a connection and understand each other on a deeper level, which is huge.

People that don't know each other very well will likely not connect like this and communicate on this deeper level. What's interesting is that even if you've only known her for 5 minutes, if you can communicate to her on this level (using socially intelligent humor, busting her balls, etc.), she'll feel like she's known you for much longer.

Mistake #9: Giving Women The Remote Control To Their Emotions

One characteristic of femininity, when looking at the female personality, is that it isn't constant—it changes like the weather does. Women tend to have more varying moods and emotional waves than men do. A mistake that I see men make is that when a woman is a bit challenging or maybe zings them with a particular comment, the man will allow that to change their mood or current state. This is one that personally took me a while to understand and get handled.

This is also one of the more advanced and challenging things you'll learn to master when gaining confidence with women.

Despite it being a slightly more advanced skill, it's still extremely important to understand and get handled as soon as you can. DO NOT let a comment, opinion, or little mood swing change your good state or mood. A woman needs to know, especially when considering you as boyfriend material, that you can handle her shit when she gets a little testy. It's your job, as a congruent, masculine man to be able to handle these moments without overreacting or letting it affect you. If you fly off the handle or get all up in arms at these moments, you're essentially acting like a little BOY. Remember, when she's acting like a little girl, YOU need to stay strong and act like the man, not the little boy. If you do, then you're both in a bad place. A woman needs a man, not a boy, always remember that.

Mistake #10: Seeing and Treating A Woman Like A Prize To Be Won Instead Of A Person

This is one that is so simple that it's easy to overlook it (or not even recognize it in the first place). It's important to constantly be reminding yourself, especially in the presence of very hot women, that they are just normal people. Under the surface of their beauty, they are no different than any other person. They have fears and insecurities; they get nervous, emotional, and self-conscious just like we men do sometimes. Remembering this will take her off the pedestal you've placed her on in your head as a result of her looks (like a prize to be won).

It's very easy to get caught up in an attractive woman's looks. Women do not have this same problem with men, at least not very often. At the end of the day, all a hot woman really wants of you is to stop showering her with affection, praise, and attention and to treat her for what she is, a human being. She'll be much more receptive to your affection, praise, and compliments if they come from a place of honesty (after you've gotten to know her a little) than she will if you say it just as fast, and in almost the same way as the last 10 guys did.

HOW TO STOP BEING SHY AND START BECOMING SUPER CONFIDENT WITH WOMEN

- **Tip 1:** "Laid Back." Even if you do not feel different in the situation, you should at least try to make it look as though you do.

Don't forget that there are many other women out there so if you lose your chances with one target, there'll be plenty more to look for. Nonetheless, if you really do have your eyes set on one target for the moment, then at least appear as though you are not overly interested in her. No woman likes a guy who comes across as obsessive and desperate.

- **Tip 2:** "Projection." Imagine yourself in a situation where you are surrounded by women. Imagine being extremely bold and having no self-confidence problems. Put yourself into this scenario and try to adapt to real life.

- **Tip 3:** "Shift of Power." Another great way to overcome self-confidence issues is to not give the woman in question the power to reject you. Going hand in hand with the first tip, you will find that if you do not come across as overly enthusiastic but just enough to engage in conversation, she will end up getting excited due to the anticipation in the air and she'll probably end up chasing you if you do things the right way.

CAN HYPNOSIS MAKE YOU MORE CONFIDENT WITH WOMEN?

Confidence is a funny old thing, and when it comes to success with women, it is incredibly important. Part of the problem is with our definition of what confidence actually is. There's the actual ability to talk and lead a conversation. If you had the knowledge and skill to be able to do this consistently then you would probably be a lot more confident. There's also the notion of self-esteem or self-worth. Men who are perceived as "confident" are usually seen as being much more attractive to women. This is much harder to fake. Anyone can learn enough lines or tricks or routines to fake knowledge, but if you truly don't believe that you deserve to be talking to this woman, then you will fail.

This is where hypnosis can help you. Everyone has elements to their personality that are attractive and elements that are unattractive. By using self-hypnosis in a clever way, you can develop more positive personality traits without any need to change "who you are." A great technique that I teach is both powerful and easy to do. It goes like this:

First, write down all the qualities you want to have when it comes to women. Describe in as much detail as possible what it will feel like when you have these qualities. You need to imagine in vivid detail how you will feel when you're chatting with women confidently.

Now make these feelings or images bigger and brighter. Step into that person and see the world through your ideal self's eyes.

Do this exercise every single day, when you're in the car, or on the train or whenever you have a free moment. The more you practice, the better you will become. The aim is to make the whole visualization process as vivid as possible.

The technique works because your subconscious mind cannot tell the difference between real and imagined events. Doing this tricks your subconscious into thinking you're having real successful encounters with women. The more vivid the imagining, the more real the subconscious will perceive it. In the same way, the subconscious mind will latch on to you imagine being rejected so don't do it!

FORGET BEING CONFIDENT WITH WOMEN, GET COMPETENT

Let's look at the definitions once again:

Confidence: full trust; belief in the powers, trustworthiness, or reliability of a person or thing: We have every confidence in their ability to succeed.

Competence: the quality of being competent; adequacy; possession of required skill, knowledge, qualification, or capacity: He hired her because of her competence as an accountant.

The former relies on belief and trust, the latter relies on demonstration and proof. It's easy to see why confidence is more appealing to men than women.

Competence requires hard work and repetition. Having information, reading books and watching videos will never replace practice. When we demonstrate competence, we express it with every part of who we are and what we do. Confidence merely creates an impression, but it lacks the substance of proof.

To move away from confidence towards competence requires action. You get competent at driving by driving. Being confident at driving without practice would be suicide. That's why we take tests, that's why we practice our swings at golf, that's why we repeat,

repeat, repeat. Repetition embeds our actions into our behavior so that it becomes second nature (competence).

So, knowing this, how can you apply it to your interactions with women? You can start by accepting that every rejection is a step closer to acceptance. Take pleasure in knowing that, repeat it to yourself before you engage in any communication with women. Rejection is feedback, it's not an attack on your personality. Imagine that you just met someone in a bar, the interaction didn't go as well as you'd like it to, she was rude to you. Is this a reflection on your personality? or hers? I may sound harsh when I say, "stop taking it personally" but this is the best advice anyone can give you. Think about it, does a tennis pro tell themselves that they are rubbish and give up if they lose a match? NO! they have lost hundreds if not thousands of matches.

Being a pro means you have failed thousands of times. Being great with women means you have had lots of rejection. Turning up to a tennis court with all the latest fashions and equipment may help you look confident, but the real measure of your ability is in your game. Get out there and play and use your feedback positively.

HOW TO TRANSFORM YOUR SELF-IMAGE WITH WOMEN!

There is a fundamental principle of the human mind I want you to really understand and incorporate, and it explains why some people really can change their lives while others just stay hoping, wishing, and stuck. It is a rule about how the human brain and mind work that controls a great deal of what we can do. And here it is:

While Your Brain May Be Attracted To Doing Something Different, Usually Brains Only DO What Is Familiar

Basically what I am saying here is, people tend to do what they are used to. People tend to think like they are used to thinking and feeling.

Yes, they may WANT to change on some level.

But the reality is, given a situation in the real world, if you are used to acting, feeling, and thinking in a certain way, just vaguely wishing you could be different ISN'T GOING TO CHANGE ANYTHING AT ALL.

The key to any kind of real change then, is mental rehearsal. You must learn to program in the way you like to feel, act, think, believe, and respond and do so with sufficient repetition that the new feelings, actions, thoughts, and beliefs are perceived by your brain as being more powerful, more vivid, more real, and more familiar Than The Way, You Used To Be!

I will say this again because it is so important. It is NOT enough to realize you want to change. It is not enough to even THINK about changing. If you want a change, especially a change that is radically different, you must Vividly, Mentally Rehearse It!

Now, I am not the first person to talk about mental rehearsal or its dirty little new age cousin, "guided visualization." The problem with most of these methods, as presented is, They Simply Do Not Work!

That's not because the people who teach or write about them don't care. It's simply because they are either leaving out vital ingredients to "make the recipe work" or because they are adding in stupid stuff that just doesn't belong.

So let me give you some vital keys to make mental rehearsal work for you, so in a matter of a few short weeks, you can totally reprogram the deepest levels of your mind for the kind of beliefs, attitudes, awareness, behaviors, and timing to bring you outrageously magnetic confidence and power with women.

- **Key #1:** The role of breath. As I pointed out last issue, breathing is of vital importance for making any deep level change.

We could get into all sorts of metaphysical explanations, but let's keep it scientific for a while at least. The scientific fact is that if you have a prolonged fear or anxiety response, eventually the limbic part of your brain that controls the flight/fight response gets progressively triggered by the smallest inputs, like a car alarm that goes off when a cat walks by.

Unless you interrupt this limbic overdrive response, any programming you try to do with the other levels of the brain and mind are going to get sabotaged and disrupted, so change will take much more "willpower" and fighting yourself.

We want to do things the easy way.

So the first step in doing your mental rehearsal for power with women will be to take ten minutes to do your breathing as taught in the previous post. And if you aren't willing to take ten minutes for yourself to succeed with women then Pack It In Now Buckwheat And Make Some More Room On The Planet!

- **Key #2:** Understanding and using the two kinds of visualization.

Anyway, there is the kind of visualization where you see yourself in the images. It's like watching a home movie of yourself, so you see your image of what you are doing or experiencing, how you are acting, etc.

This image which is useful for motivation and setting an overall direction for your mind is called disassociated. It means you are watching your self go through an experience, but you are not actually in the image, so you don't feel very much, if anything, of the feelings of being there.

THE POWER OF ASSOCIATED IMAGERY

The second kind of visualizing is where you do not see yourself in the images, but you see what you would actually see if you stepped into the image and were really there, looking out through your own eyes. We call this associated imagery, and this kind of imagery is what is most useful for fully rehearsing new behaviors, responses, emotions, and thoughts.

The key to proper mental rehearsal that really works is to first use a dissociated set of images; seeing yourself the way you would like to look, talk, and act and then switching to associated images, stepping inside the pictures and actually moving, talking, thinking, and feeling the way you'll move, talk, think, and feel when you are actually in the real situation.

Does this make sense?

First, seeing the disassociated images of the path you want to go helps to set a guidepost and a direction for your brain, so it gets an overall idea.

Then, seeing the associated images and actually walking around making the actual physical movements, talking out loud the way you'd speak, doing what you'd be actually doing FILLS IN THE DETAILS FOR YOUR BRAIN.

Before I give you this practice, remember that the process of reprogramming your subconscious mind for success with women is just that, a process. That means it takes some repetition and practice for the new thoughts, attitudes, behaviors, and feelings to take root and take hold.

So, you should practice this once a day for 2-3 weeks before you expect to see any results, though some people see results immediately.

OK then

Pick a situation—a specific context—where you'd like to have more power and confidence with women.

Let's say it is in the initial approach or walk up.

The first thing I want you to do is to sit comfortably on the flow and energize yourself with some of the breathing exercises (a key to making this work) that I've discussed before or breathing exercises you find in any good book on yoga or meditation.

The next thing I want you to do is mentally create a place in your mind where you believe anything is possible.

To do this, begin counting backward in your mind as follows:

Visualize the number 3. See it 3 times, as in 3, 3, 3. Then see the number 2, and visualize it 3 times as in 2, 2, 2. Finally, see number

1, three times as in 1, 1, 1. Mentally say each number as you see it in your mind.

Now, stand up. Imagine in front of you, a circle, on the ground. Use your actual physical arm and make the motion of drawing the circle on the ground.

Look at the circle and think of it as a place where ANYTHING can be made possible. Where anything can be made real. Where anything can be created. Then step into it.

OK. Now, imagine that situation where you want to be more confident and powerful with women. See the image of how you would look when you are that confident. See yourself acting, talking, standing, moving, and feeling as you would like to.

This is your disassociated image.

USING YOUR ASSOCIATED IMAGERY

Now, take a step forward and imagine you are actually stepping into the image so you are walking, breathing, talking from that place. See what you would actually see from your own eyes if you were there. Feel what you would feel.

Now, for an extra boost of confidence, step outside yourself and step into the woman you are meeting. Imagine you are looking at yourself through her eyes, feeling how excited she feels to meet you, hearing her voice in her head saying, "Wow...this guy is hot."

Finally, step back out of her and see your confident, powerful self again, disassociated. Mentally give yourself a command that this self will be there for you, with all the qualities, behaviors, insights, attitudes, and timing you need for total success with women.

- **Key #3** The Power Of Letting It Go

Once you've done your mental rehearsal and visualization for the day, you must dismiss it from your mind and LET IT GO.

Too often, we are taught that to get something we really want or a change we really want in ourselves, we have to constantly think about it, keeping our "goal" in the front of our mind.

In fact, this over-motivation is a load of crap that just keeps people stuck.

You have to find the proper level of motivation to create change, and that involves knowing when to just dismiss it from your mind and let it go.

It's sort of like baking cookies in an oven (here we go with baking analogies again; first it was recipes, now it's cookies!). If you put the dough in the oven but keep opening the oven door every 30 seconds to check if the cookies are done, they will never get finished!

In fact, this constant thinking if you are progressing or not or if it is working is just another form of doubt. You see, "hope" and "doubt" are really the same thing. They both involve uncertainty.

Once you've done your mental rehearsal, you need to let it go. Just release it, relax and know it will be there for you in the real world.

CHAPTER THREE

～

HAVING IRRESISTIBLE APPEAL TO WOMEN AND GETTING LAID WITH THE WOMEN OF YOUR DREAMS

If you want to attract women, you have to think like a salesman. Know what your clients want, and tune your product—that's you— to fit the clients' needs.

In order to do that, you have to do the same thing all marketers do to capture people's interest with their products: develop killer **PACKAGING**. Hey, let's face it: women judge men based on looks. And who can blame them? Before they can get to know you, they only have visual things to judge you on your clothes, your height, your body language, your status. We men are just like any other product: in order to sell well, we need great packaging!

It all comes down to women's evolutionary instincts: find the best mate for them and their unborn children. How do they do this? By seeing which men are strong, which ones are successful, and which ones have high status.

The good news is, height and wealth aren't the be-all and end-all of attraction; they're just aids to success. It's similar to saying you want a really expensive car...but that doesn't mean you'd never drive a Honda. In fact, for a lot of people (including women!), when you learn that Hondas have better mileage than Hummers, they can be more attractive! As Roberts writes, "even an ordinary man doesn't have to be exceptionally rich or powerful to make women want him. It's all a matter of the women's perspective if he ends up taller, smarter or wealthier than them."

Got that? It's all about perspective: how you market yourself successfully to a woman. Hey, lots of people know that Creative MP3 Players are better quality than iPods, but that doesn't seem to stop Apple from selling iPods like hotcakes, does it? So if you're short, or of average income, but present your positive traits in the right way, it won't matter: you'll become the iPods of men! As Roberts writes, "Think of Napoleon, Mickey Rooney or Groucho; they are humorous, artistic or politically powerful men who wooed women into their beds and, horizontally, the height issue wasn't a factor. Polite and persuasive persistence is the best trait."

So what we have are five areas that we must market effectively if we want to spark an initial attraction from women. After that, it's up to you to show what a great guy you are: let her know you're special, unique, one of a kind. That's what makes you...a best-seller!

1. Ambition

From an evolutionary standpoint, this one makes complete sense. Think cavemen and cavewomen in the Stone Age, with some of the weaker cavemen seeking a higher station in the tribe. Who do you think the cave women went for? The men who hobbled along meekly at the bottom of the order...or the men who strived for more and sought a higher place in the pack? Much of a woman's desire to be with a man who is ambitious and seeks success, is based simply on survival: The more powerful the man, the more likely she'll survive and live well. Logically, going for a guy who has no ambition means she's likely to live in poverty and struggle. Not very appealing, is it?

So you have to present yourself as a guy who's not satisfied with his station in life. This is good for both you and her. If you're making $6 an hour at McDonald's and are content to stay there, not many women are going to be attracted to you. But if you're making $6 an hour and working your ass off to own your own franchise, taking business classes at night so you can learn how to run a business: well, suddenly you're not so bad-looking! Believe me, women will give men a chance, they want to give men a chance—as long as they see potential. Know that quote, "Behind every great man is an even greater woman"? Show you've got potential and direction, and you'll get that great woman.

2. Status

Again, evolutionary instincts of survival make women naturally attracted to men of high status. High status equals good living for herself and her children. Fortunately, projecting high status does not have to be difficult; according to Roberts, "Wearing the right clothes, especially nice shoes, can go a long way toward portraying wealth. Taking on the unshaken or unworried attitude of wealthy men can project affluence. Hesitant, irresolute, bland men come across as having lower incomes and being less reliable." Got that? You don't have to be a powerful, articulate man yourself—you just have to project similar qualities.

SOME OF THESE QUALITIES INCLUDE:

- **Not Putting Yourself Down.** Without being a braggart, talk positively about your accomplishments, job position, and possessions—even if they're not much. If you treat things as a big deal, other people will, too. Conversely, if you downplay your accomplishments and character, women will too. Your attitude is contagious, so make sure it's an enthusiastic, enlivening one that people enjoy.

- **Act Like You Deserve Good Women.** Don't let women assume a higher status than you. Show them that YOU are the one with higher status. You can do this in a number of ways, including not acting impressed by a woman's beauty or career (say, she's a model), teasing her about her clothes or makeup, and asking her to buy you a drink. Chances are she won't, but just by acting like you deserve it, you raise your status! She's not such an untouchable goddess in the end.

Remember, as well, that women want to EARN a man; they relish the challenge of luring in a winning catch. So play hard to get: talk to other girls, say you've got to be leaving just when things are going well, don't immediately ask for her phone number. If you act like a man who can have his pick of women, then chances are, you will!

- **Knowing People Of High Status.** This is a great one. Get to know the people of power: the club owners, bartenders, maitre'ds. Position yourself as a sociable person who's in the knows. When a woman sees you getting special treatment and chatting with high-status people, she'll see right away that you're someone of importance. It will also reduce the importance of the other factors, such as height, money, and ambition; immediately you've proven yourself valuable.

- **Social Proof/Female Acquaintances.** Hey, nothing says, "This guy's attractive" than having females around him. Of course, the hotter they are, the hotter you look, but even just having an average-looking female's company can only help: it shows women that other women are interested in you. Do your best to get your female friends and family (sisters, cousins) to come out with you. It's social proof, and it works!

- **Wearing Nice Clothes.** "When a man is well dressed," writes communications expert Leil Lowndes, "it signifies his ability to provide for her offspring." You don't have to be rich and powerful to wear nice clothes. You just have to show that you're a man of quality, a man headed somewhere who pays attention to dress (something women can never get enough of). Formal clothes, such as a suit, convey that you are serious about success; you desire good things. So just by wearing a nice sports jacket, dress shirt, and slacks, you let a woman know you're a man with status. You're a man who could provide for her and her children.

The colors you wear are vital: Studies show that red, burgundy, and black clothes convey high status. So get yourself some slick black suits or formal wear, a redshirt, and one of my favorites (and girls'!), a sleek burgundy button-down shirt. They all convey regality and strength.

In the case of red, you have the added bonus of sexuality, power, and dominance: definitely good qualities to portray! Go and purchase a nice red polo shirt or red tie for your suit.

If you enjoy white clothes—the color of purity and cleanliness—then make sure you work on your TAN. White clothes against a dark backdrop make you look exotic, sexy, and well-traveled. You don't have to be a jet-setting playboy to look like one!

- **Winning Body Language.** Women judge men by the way they move and position themselves; it's part of their superior communication skills to know what a man is thinking or feeling based on his body language. So, position yourself in the right way: don't slouch, sit upright, gaze at her knowingly, lean into her to initiate intimacy. I've got a great column on body language that will teach you the right ways and the wrong ways to project high status.

3. Financial Resources

According to Matthew Fitzgerald, "Studies with college coeds show that when shown photographs of men dressed in high-status uniforms, ties, expensive watches, etc.) and low-status uniforms, these women would be significantly more willing to enter into relationships with the more expensively-attired males regardless of the man's physical appearance. To a woman, attraction is simple: green is very good-looking."

Okay, so not every guy has money for expensive suits and watches, and materialism may not be part of your game. However, if you want to impress women, one of the fastest ways is by wearing snazzy clothes, sporting nice shoes (girls LOVE shoes!), and driving an expensive car. Especially when it comes to designer brands, women are VERY keen at spotting high-quality products. It's just part of their nature; with expensive possessions come high status and ambition, and a more comfortable lifestyle. Again, this all comes from their instinctual drive for survival and prosperity for themselves and their children. By owning the best, you become the best. At least on the surface.

Ultimately, if you want true love it's up to you to find women who share the same goals and values. If money and status aren't the most important things in life for you, don't chase the girls who prioritize those things. Don't go for the shallow, bitchy types who only judge a man by how much he can spend on her.

4. Educational Level

Knowledge really is power, and on top of that, it's an aphrodisiac! Gone are the days when being smart was acquainted with being a nerd; now, knowledge and intelligence are your friends. It's the easiest way to money and the easiest way to success. So show it off a little. Let her know your TALENTS, your interests, your areas of special knowledge. As Roberts writes, "Women are drawn to experts like the Crocodile Hunter, Bill Gates, and Chris Rock because they're experts in their industries." None of those guys are particularly good-looking, but they're good at what they do, and parlay their knowledge into success, which drives women wild.

A guy who's an expert is one who is clearly successful and of higher status. At the very least, having a special type of knowledge means you have the TOOLS for success and can provide intellectual stimulation for a girl (which, unless she's a bimbo with an IQ of 70, is quite important for women).

Additionally, just being in school is a great way to show off your knowledge: "If you're in school, not only are there more women available, but you've already demonstrated to them that you're getting educated. Otherwise, it's up to you to come across as reliable and credible without making her feel dumb."

5. Physical Aptitude

Physical height alone is an easy way to catch a woman's attention, but it's not the only thing. Again, evolutionary mechanics come into play here. A man who is tall, strong, and athletic is more likely to fend off threats to the woman and her children. He is also more likely to have a strong immune system, which will further aid their chances of survival. So, you can't blame women too much for valuing these things: in the world of female attraction, it really is the survival of the fittest. Those who show women they are in shape and healthy are much more likely to survive the dating game! Ergo, athletes, bouncers, firemen get the girls.

As for height, it's all a matter of perspective. We've all seen short guys with tall beautiful women. Neil Strauss himself, the best of the best pickup artists, is just 5'6" yet gets more beautiful women than we can imagine. How? By believing in himself. By positioning himself as a man of high status. By not bowing down to women of greater height or beauty. And by being a guy women know it is fun to be around. In short, he's got INNER GAME, and when you have that down, nothing can stop you. You may even find yourself dating women who are taller than you!

CHAPTER FOUR

❦

HOW TO MEET WOMEN, ANYTIME, ANYWHERE

You should talk to women just as you would talk to anyone else. That's because women actually are anyone else. They are just people like you and me. Even the most beautiful woman is just a regular person with the same basic wants and needs as everyone else. Usually, the problem with talking to women is that we clam up, or that we put them on such a pedestal that we make ourselves look subservient and weak. If you have had trouble talking to women, then this chapter will cover a few things that you will need to know so that you don't make the mistake of talking yourself out of a good situation.

Be unconcerned with approval. In general, women are attracted to men who have some clear goals and know that they are on the road to achieving them. One way to signal this type of attitude is to abandon approval-seeking conversations in favor of bold, confident talk. This does not mean being boorish, ignoring the other people in the conversation and hogging the woman's speaking time. Rather, you should speak your mind confidently and clearly. If people laugh at you don't suddenly change your tune to agree with them. Also, avoid sycophantic confirmation of the statements of other people. If someone (especially the woman you want to attract) says something you disagree with, just say so. Not in a rude way, but as any well-adjusted adult should be able to do.

Express romantic interest. Keeping in line with the idea of being confident and goal-directed, if you are romantically interested in a woman (and that's what this is all about, right?) don't be afraid to tell her about it. Hiding behind platitudes and feigned friendliness is obvious falsity; you didn't approach a woman in a nightclub because you wanted someone to play checkers with. She will respect your honesty.

If she is not interested in you, she will just say so, freeing you up to move along to a more receptive woman. Again, this does not mean you should use crass or blunt language, just that you should clearly express your interest with your words.

Point out positives along with the negatives. While you are talking to a woman there is sometimes the urge to shower her with compliments. She may well deserve them, but chances are she has been bombarded with this type of conversation since she was a teenager. It's fine to compliment her, but you can also point out some of her faults, too. If she has an ugly dress on, tell her. Just make sure to phrase it in a joking, playful manner. Let her know you dislike her clothes, but that you aren't pointing it out just to be a jerk. Again, she will respect your honesty.

The best way to talk to a woman is with honesty, directness, and confidence. Tell her what you really think and she will be able to accept or reject you based on who you actually are. And if you talk to her that way, chances are it will be the former.

Perfect Cure for Starting a Conversation With a Woman

I have a simple 2-step formula that will end all of your worries.

That formula is: **Observe, then Question.**

Allow me to explain:

- **Step 1** – Observe – You must become observant when you are out. Not only will it increase your ability to drive a conversation, but it will also enhance your life and help you to notice things most people never do.

When you become observant, you begin to notice small things about her that most men don't. When creating that first impression and building rapport with her, setting yourself apart from every other guy is ESSENTIAL! If she thinks you're different, she will let you stay.

Here's a little secret. Women do their hair, nails, makeup, match their outfits to their purses, etc., for two reasons. They want to look nice and they want to feel nice. If they feel like they look nice, they feel good. If they feel good, men will talk to them.

So – women make themselves look nice so men notice! It's that simple. But, sadly, most men never do.

Observe things about her – her hair, nails, eye makeup, blouse, body language, does she appear to be waiting for someone, these are what will drive your future conversation.

Observe your surroundings. Things that may be going on around you, temperature, smells, weird people, is there a guy talking to her? Maybe by her body language you perceive she is not interested (Good approach: you sit down next to her and pretend like you've known her a long time. When he leaves, tell her she looked like she needed help, then continue talking).

- **Step 2** - Question. You can control an entire conversation just by asking open-ended conversation (not interview-style) questions. You just start asking questions based on your observations, wait for her answer, elaborate, and take that topic as far as it will go. If it leads to another topic, great! If you have "dead air" just ask about another observation you made.

EX: "Hey, I like your shoes by the way. Where would I be able to get a pair of them for my sister as a birthday present?

HOW TO FLIRT WITH A GIRL THAT YOU ARE ATTRACTED TO

It is always recommended to start out with small talk with a girl you like. Chat with her about common matters, studies, her friends, her family, and her interests. Do not rush her. Stay calm and composed with her. Do not flood her with compliments. She might think you are faking it. Always focus your actions on starting from a nice acquaintance to intimate friendship to love and desire.

1.   **Start with the humor! Learn to be witty try and throw out some jokes.**

This will help make her comfortable in her interactions with you. Most of the girl's align intelligence and confidence together. So make her believe that you stick to your word and that you are secure with yourself. If you say something that doesn't come off quite right, follow it up with something funny and turn it into a joke.

2.   **The Next Step In Flirting With A Girl Is Being Confident.**

Flirting with a woman that you are interested in, can be done using your body language. Body language is an essential but often overlooked part of communication. Not only your body gestures but also the dressing style can be vital while flirting

3.   Flirting Means Sitting Close To Her And Not Breathing Down Her Neck.

Two chairs side-by-side is just what is exactly needed for that moment. Never be too eager to start up a conversation. Give her the opportunity as well. Tell her a short story if there is a long pause between your talks. Be a good listener too.

4.   Find Out Her Interests Like The Music She Likes, Authors She Reads, Etc.

Talk to her about these things. If you can't think of anything to talk about, start the conversation using a starter like "How has your day been?"

5.   Praise Also Plays An Important Role.

A woman's beauty is her asset. More often than not, when she wants to get a man's attention, she will show it off. So praise her but don't overdo it! She will take your flirtation to a higher level if she is serious about you. This should be taken as a gesture of acceptance of your flirtation.

6.   You Can Also Start Flirting With Gifts.

Be patient with your lady love. Try giving her little gifts like a yellow rose and gradually a red rose. Stuffed animals are often preferred by the girls. A small cup of coffee can also work wonders in your efforts to flirt.

7.   Another Good Way To Flirt Is To Give Her A Shoulder To Cry Upon.

Don't make her cry, but if she feels like telling you some sad things from throughout her life, be a sport and console her. Try to help her out with problems. Do not interfere too much. She will come to you when ready. Reassure her that you are always there for her. You can always spice up her mood by starting a surprising conversation that she might not be expecting.

8.   Play Small Games Like Eye Contact

Once you are glued to her eyes, you can always find out whether she has any interest in you. When you approach a woman, always pay attention to her eyebrows. If they are immediately raised but are followed by steady eye contact and a smile, you have probably got the green signal to proceed.

HOW TO GET DATES WITH WOMEN EASILY

1.   Be Witty.

You should be able to converse with them. You need to use your brain and wits. They are intimidating. You just need to focus on getting a good conversation with them. You need to impress them with your wits. You need to make them feel that you are not intimidated by them. You need to make a good impression. If you feel that she's smart, you have to read more. You have to know more. You have to read books that she's into. That way, when she asks you a question, you know what to say.

2.   Build Up That Confidence.

Don't get eaten up by your insecurities. You need to boost your self-esteem. Now, how do you get yourself to do that? It's simple. You can start by learning to appreciate yourself. You can list out all the good qualities that you have. You will begin to realize that you have a lot of things to offer. Remember, your insecurities will show in the way you walk, stand, sit, and talk. When you slouch, it shows that you are not happy with your own self. You need to make it a point to boost your ego once in awhile. You can begin by doing the things that you love.

3.   Be The Casanova.

You can be the gentleman that they have been longing for. When you see her, don't tell her that she's beautiful. Tell her something distinct and that she hasn't heard before. Compliment her attitude. She will think that you don't go for her looks and body. Also, you can offer to drive her to her house. It would be a sweet thing of you to do. You can do things that can knock her feet off the ground.

4.   When All Else Fails, Do The Opposite.

Yes, it is ironic. But perhaps, the goody-two-shoes doesn't work for her. You can be the bad boy or that obnoxious guy she gets irritated with. It takes a lot of guts to try this because some men fail at this.

You can be superficially mean to her. You can superior to her. Maybe that is what she needs. She needs someone who is better than her and someone who is not threatened by her.

HOW TO SEDUCE A WOMAN WITHOUT TOUCHING HER

1.   Speak Like A Detective.

One of the first things you need to realize is that you embody your status to the world through your voice. It is extremely important for you to enhance the power of your voice in order to seduce a woman without touching her.

"Never raise your voice at the end of your sentence while talking." Make your voice low at the end of sentences. When you end sentences smoothly, you automatically project your authority and lead her mental state with your dominance. This is the secret of detectives that makes girls shiver. In addition, vampires also speak like detectives and end their sentences on low voice. That's why vampires are also extremely seductive for women.

2.   Anklets Are Highly Erotic For A Woman.

There is no doubt that anklets keep a woman erotic throughout the day. Gift her anklets in order to arouse her sexual emotions for you. Anklets won't only keep her erotic but also make her think about you all day. Anklets are one of the best ways to seduce a woman without touching her.

3.   Make Her Wear Red Color.

Red color biologically appeals to almost everyone. A woman feels immensely energetic after wearing a red color dress because it is a color of love.

For arousing her sexual feelings, ask your woman to wear a red color dress. You can gift her some red lingerie or a red bikini. Even the most prudish woman can be seduced rather easily with a red color dress/gift because the color red stimulates the sexual feelings of a woman and transforms her into a seductive lady.

4.   Be A Handyman.

It becomes easier to seduce a woman when you act like a handyman. Most men rely on others instead of taking action with their own hands. They become unable to do their own integral things. Therefore, women often avoid being with them.

On the other hand, a handyman creates sexual energy because of his action taking habit. He fixes something at his home, washes his car, cooks special dishes, mows the lawn, makes coffee, etc. He loves taking action, and he projects his masculinity. A woman feels positive sexual energy in the presence of a handyman.

5.   Dominate Her Mind.

One way to seduce a woman without touching her is to dominate her mind. Women have been attracted to men that dominate their minds, make them laugh, and share interesting stories. If you desire to dominate a woman's mind utterly, then you should learn the art of storytelling.

"THE COMBINATION OF CURIOSITY AND FUN IN YOUR CONVERSATION AROUSES SEXUAL FEELINGS OF A WOMAN."

In order to arouse sexual feelings of a woman, make her laugh with your stories, stimulate her mind with curiosity and stay original. When you make a girl laugh while keeping the curiosity alive through your stories, you easily arouse her sexual feelings for you.

Remember, you may end up yourself into her friend category if you don't generate curiosity. Curiosity is essential for keeping women on their toes all the time.

Boys make women laugh. On the other hand, adults arouse the sexual feelings of women with curiosity and fun.

6.   Seductive Body Language.

A woman can immediately recognize your body language. Most of the advice preaches about basic body language but a woman notices you in great detail. It is very tough for an average man to hide his actual persona and project seductive body language.

If you want to seduce a woman with your seductive body language then here I am giving you few tips which will help you a lot of your entire life.

- Never nod your head rapidly. It is a sign of eagerness and impatience. You project yourself like an impatient boy instead of an actual masculine man.

- Keep your eyebrows relaxed. When you show confident body language, you often forget to relax your eyebrows. When a woman looks at your raising eyebrows, she immediately understands that you are not comfortable and trying to hide your inner excitement.

- Your facial expressions highly attract women. Have you ever thought why Johnny Depp is extremely attractive to women? It is because he has an artistic face and he makes women melt with his facial expressions. Your eyebrows are integral for making your expressions attractive. So, set your eyebrows and correct your expressions in order to seduce a woman.

HOW TO TOUCH A WOMAN FROM THE MOMENT YOU FIRST MEET HER TO THE MOMENT YOU TWO GET SEXUAL

When learning how to touch a woman, you should focus on the following two important things: first off, you always be totally comfortable with touching women, and second off, you have to make sure that whenever you touch a woman, she feels completely comfortable with you touching her.

The key to understanding these two vital things is that when you touch a woman and she realizes that touching her feels totally natural and fun to you, not only will she start to trust you more but she'll also start to feel very comfortable with touching you back. The reason why she'll trust you more is because it's well tested and proven that whenever you do or say something that feels totally natural and fun to you while meeting a woman, it's very likely that she'll soon start to subconsciously see you as an authority or an expert on the thing that you're doing or saying to her.

Once you get her to feel comfortable with you touching her, all you should be doing next is use the right type of touch that matches the right mindset that you should embrace at each one of the three different stages of interaction: attraction, rapport, and seduction. Next, I'm going to share with you the 3 steps on how to touch a woman from the moment you first meet her to the moment you two get sexual.

1. Use Your Hand Gestures To Bridge The Gap Between Not Touching Her And Starting To Touch Her

When learning how to touch a woman at the very beginning of an interaction, you should make sure that you do the following two vital things: first off, you need to learn how to use your hand gestures without touching the woman in order to bridge the gap between not touching her and touching her, and second off, you need to learn how to properly touch her without freaking her out. Next, I'm going to give you the step-by-step instructions on how to smoothly transition from not touching her into starting to touch her.

Before you start touching the woman that you've just met, you always need to make sure that she feels totally comfortable with you touching her.

The safest way to bridge the gap between not touching her at all and starting to touch her is to use your hand gestures. Using your hand gestures will basically help you overcome any of the woman's initial touching barriers.

Your hand gestures are meant to help you smoothly enter her personal space without touching her yet on one hand, and on the other hand, they're meant to help you indirectly let her know that you might be touching her very soon. Once she feels comfortable with you invading her personal space without touching her yet, then you can move straight to touching her.

So, here's what you do. While you're talking to the woman, try to slightly move one of your hands around her so that you can easily enter her touch zone. You just make the motion of touching her without actually touching her. You just move your hand right near her as if you're going to touch her. You want to move it slowly because if you move it too fast, she's going to flinch and feel like she needs to protect herself. I suggest that you make that hand motion as many times as necessary until you notice that she feels totally comfortable with it. Once you see that she's completely comfortable with your hand gestures, you can then start touching her.

I'm going to show you how to touch a woman at each one of the three different stages of interaction: attraction, rapport, and seduction.

2. Touch Her Playfully For A Couple Of Seconds At The Stage Of Attraction.

When touching the woman at the stage of attraction, you have to make sure that your touch lasts for no longer than 1-3 seconds. This is why some top seducers like to call this type of touch a temporary touch. At the stage of attraction, your touch must feel very playful and lighthearted on her skin because you want to get her attracted to you by touching her in a way that shows her that you might be potentially interested in her while not being needy towards her. This is why it's extremely important that at this point you embrace your playful mindset.

The parts of the woman's body that are considered appropriate to touch at the stage of attraction are her upper outer arm, her shoulders, and her upper back. For example, you could put your arm around her shoulder as if she's your friend. But make sure that you don't put your arm around her neck because most women aren't comfortable with that.

3. Touch her softly and caringly for 3-5 seconds at the stage of rapport while pretending to be her best friend.

You should embrace the mindset of being the woman's best friend when touching her at the stage of rapport because you want to build trust and comfort with her. Here you have to forget and let go of that playful mindset that you had at the attraction stage. You also have to make sure that you're not rushing your mind into thinking of having sex with the woman when you're at the stage of rapport. You want to come across as a non-wanting and non-needy man who's not desperate to get anything out of her. What you want to focus on at this point is simply getting to know her.

During the stage of rapport, you want to be touching her as if you want to share with her something that you normally don't share with anybody else. You also want to be prepared to kind of console her if she's feeling sad or having a hard time with something. You need to make her feel accepted through showing her that you totally understand her and her current situation in life. Even if she says to you that she likes to kick her little puppies sometimes, you should just show her that you understand that.

The kind of touch that you should use during the rapport stage is a lingering touch. This type of touch lasts for about 3-5 seconds. At this point, your touch should feel very soft and caring.

The woman's body parts that are considered appropriate to touch at the stage of rapport are her hands, her low back, and her face.

Here's a little sign of warning. When touching the woman's hands, you should touch them for 3-5 seconds but without holding them.

The reason why you should be touching the woman for no longer than 5 seconds during the stage of rapport is because you want to get her to want you to touch her more. This touching strategy basically helps you warm her up and get her ready for entering the seduction stage without giving you any kind of her resistance later.

The way you'd touch her during the stage of rapport is that, for example, you'd slightly push and brush her hair out of her face. You could also touch the back of her neck and kind of slide your fingers slowly up the back of her head. This touching technique is proven successful when transitioning from the stage of rapport to the stage of seduction.

The way you can initiate the above touching technique is by simply saying to the woman something like: "Let me try this real quick and see how it feels." Then, you simply put one of your hands at the bottom of the back of her neck and ride it up her neck so that your fingers are facing the top of her head. So, you'd run your fingers up her neck as if you were going to grab her hair. And, then at the root of her hair, you'd grab a handful of her hair. Next, you'd simply pull her head back and down slowly so that she has to pull it up.

Here's an important warning. I strongly advise you that you only do the whole hair grabbing and hair pulling thing at the tail-end of the stage of rapport.

4. **Touch her powerfully but still caringly for as long as you want during the stage of seduction.**

During the stage of seduction, you should be touching her in a way that shows her that you're a powerful man. Your touch should feel powerful and manly but still caring because you never want to be hurting her. The way to make sure that you don't hurt her is to use a little bit of your playfulness and then mix it up with your manly power. But also make sure that you never snap out of your overall sexual state at this stage because if you do, the woman will soon snap out of her sexual state too and the game will be over.

At the stage of seduction, you want to make sure that you touch her in a very sexual way. Your touch should feel very desiring to the woman because you want to make her feel desired.

During the stage of seduction, you should use a constant touch. The constant touch means that you can keep your touch on one part of her body for as long as you want.

Your touch should feel not only very powerful and manly but also very palm heavy. What I mean by the word "palm heavy" is that if you, for example, want to move from touching her low back to touching her legs, you should just keep dragging or sliding your hand's palm from her low back area over her ass area all the way down to her legs area. In other words, you don't need to take your hand off her low back in order to move it and then put it on her legs or any other area of her body that you want to touch next.

The reason why you should never lift up your hand when wanting to move from touching one area of her body to touching another area of her body is because if you do, you face the risk of having her completely snap out of her sexual state. If she snaps out of her sexual state, the game will be over. This is why it's extremely important that you use a palm heavy touch during the stage of seduction.

Here's an important note. Make sure that you never apologize to the woman for touching her in a certain way if you've touched her the right way and at the right time during an interaction. The reason why I strongly advise you not to apologize to her for it is because if you do, not only will she subconsciously see you as a very insecure and creepy guy but also she might fiercely reject you.

Here's why she sees your apologizing as a big turn-off: whenever you apologize to the woman for something that you don't need to apologize for, she'll instantly see you as a very weak man who's unsure of himself and his feelings.

As for the woman's body areas that are considered appropriate to touch at the stage of seduction, it's needless to say that you can be touching any part of her body at this point as long as you're not hurting her in any way.

CHAPTER FIVE

❦

HOW TO GET A WOMAN TO BED

SIGNS SHE'S HOT FOR YOU

A woman is full of mystery and the more you try to decode her hidden moves, the more complicated things become. If you want to skip the hard parts in your pursuit of a woman, you need to learn how to read her body language and finally get to know what she really means without her saying what she really means straight to your face and of course, you will definitely get her to notice you more than the rest. Below are the five signs she's hot for you—use them to find out if she wants to sleep with you tonight!

- **She Makes The Moves On You**. She flirts alright, but it's different when a woman is already actually hitting on you. Try to figure it out by the way she acts. It's like she just can't wait for you to make the moves anymore. She's trying to give you hints on what she wants to tell you but she just can't spill it out. Hey, what more can you ask for!!! All you have to do is make things just right for both of you.

- **She's In A More Hyper Mood**. You might say that when you hit her with humor, she actually laughs out loud or she's speaking her mind in an aggressive way. If she's obviously in a much happier mood when you're around, it simply means that seeing you makes her feel good.

- **She Gets A Little Too Close For Comfort**. She reaches over and touches you briefly but constantly. A woman who's turned on will try to initiate a little bit of intimacy and observes how you react. You need to observe her body language and finally find out if she wants some real action tonight.

- **She Teases And Gets Playful**. It's like she wants to hug you but somehow tries it in another way and she wants you to do exactly the same with her! You know it when a girl is on the mood for something else rather than plain flirting— when she gets all rowdy and jumpy, she might want to get to bed sooner than you expect it.

- **She Shows You She's Interested**. You know it based on how she reacts to the things you tell her. When she asks a lot of questions, she's somewhat curious and interested in knowing you better. Hey, if someone doesn't like you, why bother, right? If she checks on you frequently and wants to hang out with you most of the time or she canceled some of her appointments just for you, then she's definitely interested.

HOW TO START A SEXUAL CONVERSATION WITH A GIRL WITHOUT SOUNDING AWKWARD OR CREEPY

The goal here is to introduce sexual tension and generate attraction with her.

Truth is, if you keep talking to a girl you're interested in on the level of a friend, she will categorize you as a friend in her mind.

She will see you as just a friend, but not someone she feels sexually attracted to.

Now, the drawback to this is that women or girls know that men want to have sex with them. So any tentative suggestion or advances from you can cause a woman to raise her defenses.

So how do you go about this? How do you start a sexual conversation with a girl without raising any red flags?

Exactly as the title says, in this article I teach you how to start a sexual conversation with a girl without sounding awkward or creepy.

You'll learn the 3 best ways to introduce the topic of sex without telegraphing your interest.

Before You Begin...

Know that women love to talk about sex...

But most of them are reluctant to talk about it with men they don't feel comfortable with or don't have an emotional connection with.

So before you initiate sexual topics with a woman or a girl, make sure you've gained rapport with her first.

It's even better if she's giving you some indications of interest. For instance, when she's playing with her hair, touching you, or leaning in close when conversing.

With that said, let's get started... on how to start a sexual conversation with a girl.

Here's How To Start A Sexual Conversation With A Girl:

- **Tip #1:** Talk about things from the sexual perspective

Let's say you're talking about a movie.

Don't tell her how much you liked it for its car chase and how some dude got to kick some more ass.

Instead, tell her about how you liked the love relationship between the characters.

And how you loved the sensuality of their scenes together. And then you ask her if there are any other movies that have affected her that way and have her explain why.

- **Tip #2:** Feed her mind

Slip in sexually charged words or phrases into your normal conversation with her.

A great way to do this is by using sexual innuendos or double entendre. This is when you say something innocent, yet can be deemed dirty or sexual.

For instance:

> "Boy, this is really hard." (When you're talking about a popsicle.)

> "I didn't come with her." (When you're talking about a party you went to.)

> "He almost rear-ended her." (When you're talking someone getting hit by a car.)

Another effective way to feed her mind or gradually bring up sexual topics is to use "That's what she said jokes" and "That's what he said jokes."

When she says something like:

"Put it inside"

"It's much better when it's wet"

"Do you want to come inside" (when she's inviting you into her apartment)

then you respond with:

"T'at's what SHE said"

Or when she says something like...

"'ou're making it hard (for me)"

'It's getting really hard"

"I want to eat the whole thing"

then you respond with:

"T'at's what HE said"

When she says something dirty on purpose, then tease her for having a dirty mind.

Of course, you 'on't want to go into this territory during the early stages or when 'ou've just met.

You start with superficial conversation, then build it up to a more sexual conversation.

Again, make sure 'ou've gained rapport with her first. Then you start using words that are sexually charged in your conversation.

And with time, 'he'll be comfortable talking about sexual topics with you.

If she do'sn't play along, then she probably 'sn't comfortable with you yet.

Next on how to start a sex conversation with a girl...

- **Tip #3:** Bring up a sexual situation of a friend of yours

For instance:

You can tell her you have a female friend who is complaining that her boyfriend do'sn't like going down south during sex. And she thinks her boyfriend do'sn't like the idea of going down on her or 'sn't taking the hints he's giving him.

Now, ask her how women can suggest things like that to their men.

"So how do women hint at that sort of thing?"

(You see what you're doing here... you're getting her to specifically talk about sex)

Now, if she talks freely on the subject of sex, then she's comfortable discussing sexual situations with you.

And from here on, she'll start initiating sexual conversations with you.

So there you have it... how to start a sex conversation with a girl or a woman.

Understand this: Don't make the girl or woman you're talking to the subject of sexual conversation. Only talk about other people's sexual situations.

TOP WAYS TO BOOST YOUR SEXUAL CONFIDENCE WITH WOMEN

- **Uncover The Source Of Sexual Confidence**

Sexual Confidence comes as a result of knowing how to give a woman mind-blowing pleasure. It's the confidence that the woman you're with will have a once-in-a-lifetime experience with you. It's knowing all the steps—from the first eye contact all the way to the "end game"—and knowing how to build ANTICIPATION every step along the way. Start by practicing my "two steps forward, one step back" technique by escalating things, then backing off, then escalating further, then backing off again. The anticipation and arousal this creates will drive her INSANE. Don't say I didn't warn you.

- **Get Out Of The Manipulation Mindset**

Guys are always curious about how to "trick" a girl into bed—what the magic words are, etc. I personally know a few guys who do this... and I can tell you it does NOT lead to fulfillment. Avoid this whole "manipulation mindset," and stop trying to figure out what the magic bullets are to get a woman to do what you want in a dishonest way. It's much better to work on becoming an interesting guy who knows what to do to build attraction in a natural, nonmanipulative way. If what you're doing feels wrong or unethical, stop it. There are better ways to get what you want.

- **Stop Idealizing Beautiful Women**

Most guys get fooled into believing that just because a woman is unusually attractive, she's also usually honest and would never consider taking from you, cheating on you or lying to you. The reality is that people are never 100% "good" or 100% "bad." There are situations where ANY person would lie, cheat, steal, or be disloyal. When you accept the reality that people are people, a beautiful woman is still human, and that the woman you feel strongly for is just as likely to be dishonest or disloyal as any other, you'll take her off that pedestal you put her on. And that's an important step toward achieving sexual confidence.

How Important Are Looks When It Comes To Being Confident In Bed?

- **Looks Don't Matter When It Comes To Sexual Confidence**

Nothing about how you look, how old you are, how tall you are, how much you weigh, how much money you make, or whether or not you're her type has ANYTHING to do with how you can make a woman feel once you're in bed with her. A key to remember is that AFTER a woman has experienced a mind-blowing intimate experience with you, that experience alone will render all of that other stuff irrelevant. It just won't matter. Picture yourself in this future ahead of time and it'll help make it a self-fulfilling prophecy.

- **Delay Your Gratification**

Delaying gratification becomes more profound the more you think about it—and when it comes to sex, it's absolutely critical. It not only allows you to build the sexual tension and make her want you more and more, but the teasing and anticipation act as amplifiers to HER arousal. Bottom line: You are more likely to turn her on— and more likely to take things to a physical level—if you're cool and calm. Lose your need for instant results, and you'll drive her CRAZY.

- **Act Like Sex Is Normal**

A lot of guys get nervous when it comes time to have sex; they think they need to start acting differently when it's time to "do the deed." But sex is normal, so keep acting normal as things heat up. Don't make a big deal out of it; keep having fun; keep teasing; keep acting light. Smoothly, confidently, comfortably progress from one step to the next, all the while enjoying yourself and acting like all is normal—because it is.

- **Put Sex Into Perspective**

Instead of positioning sex as the ultimate goal and the center of your purpose, move it so it's simply one of your many goals. Make it a natural outcome if you like a woman and if you choose to spend the time and effort to get to that point. Take the "pinnacle value" out of sex, put it in perspective, and your relaxed attitude will make you much more likely to get it.

- **Tame The Fear Of Rejection**

As you progress from one step to the next with a woman—from a casual date to touching, kissing and beyond—the stakes get bigger and bigger. Men typically feel more apprehensive as they progress from one step to the next, and feel less confident moving to the next step as things get more intense. The fear is not of being rejected or stopped, but of losing all the ground that has been gained, and going back to ZERO. Fortunately, the more involved you get, the more likely it is you'll succeed. The next step involves less risk, and it makes the sexual act more likely. Remember this.

- **Interpret Her Actions**

If she stops you, it usually doesn't mean that she wants you to stop FOREVER; it means that you didn't get her turned on enough. Interpret it as "I'm not ready yet," rather than "Go away, I don't like you anymore." Stop, lean back, talk casually for a while and just relax. Then get her even MORE turned on than before. Feel free to make her ASK you for sex... or even beg. "Please" is a great word— teach her to use it, and she'll LOVE you for it.

- **Get In Touch With The Animal Inside**

A woman wants a man who's in touch with his inner ANIMAL. If he's overly logical, overly analytical, overly controlled, overly educated, then it shows a woman that he cannot let the animal out. At an instinctive level, a woman knows that this means she won't be able to FEEL anything strong toward him, and she knows he won't be able to arouse any sexual feelings inside of her. Study, get to know, make friends with, and DEVELOP the animal inside you. Educating yourself in this area is one of the most important things you can do to take your sexual confidence to the next level.

THE BEST WAY TO GET A WOMAN IN BED AND MAKE A WOMAN WANT YOU

Any healthy, loving, and lasting relationship counts a great sex life as a key ingredient. And if you look around you, it's probably not hard to tell which couples are truly happy with each other. These are the couples that still look at each other with lust in their eyes! So what's their secret? It's probably that they are BOTH sexually satisfied in their relationship.

A lot of people know that women don't reach orgasm as easily or as quickly as men. What many don't realize is that this does nothing but build sexual frustration, which is one of the common female problems. And sexual frustration manifests itself in many negative ways in a relationship; until one day, you both wake up and realize that you no longer have passion for each other or in your lives. By then, even satibo capsules will not help to ignite the passion.

The good news is it's really not hard at all to make a woman reach an orgasm. But you both have to work at it, which, if you think about it, is part of the fun as well!

You may find this step-by-step guide useful. It is one of the many tools that Gabrielle Moore, an expert on sex education has created.

STEP 1

Engage in a lot of foreplay! Foreplay is very important because it helps her relax her mind and makes her more focus on the lovemaking at hand. It is a much-needed female orgasm enhancer. It's also a great way to bond as many women associate foreplay as a man's way of taking time and ensuring sex is not just a physical act but about intimacy.

Foreplay can start hours or even days in advance and is really limited only by your sexual imagination. As you keep this "sexual tension" high, you'll find that it's actually easier to bring her to orgasm once you do engage in sex.

STEP 2

If foreplay is the "primer," oral sex is the next big step. Many women actually claim that oral sex is the ONLY way they can reach an orgasm, so if you want to make sure she reaches climax, then don't resist.

When you do go down on her, don't rush it. Show her that you really love her by lavishing her with your undivided attention. Enjoy the journey as much as the destination so to speak.

At the start, just tease and lick softly and lovingly. Once she's focused on that part of her body, increase the tempo. When you notice that her breathing is getting faster and harder or if her legs are becoming taut, move your attention to her clitoris. Tease it by drawing small circles around it with your tongue and then apply more pressure and lick faster.

If she gives any indication at all that she's really turned on, remember this: DON'T change anything. Keep the tempo of what you're doing and she'll reach her orgasm soon enough.

STEP 3

If your tongue doesn't bring her to an immediate orgasm, don't despair. Don't forget that your fingers can be put to good use too! Use your index finger to "trace" the outline of her labia. Be sure to touch her gently. This is guaranteed to electrify her body. After this, place your index and middle finger together and then draw circles around her clitoris.

Pay attention to her body (is it in a pleasured, relaxed state or is it pulled taut like a string?) to gauge just how turned on she is. Don't forget to pay attention to her moans and groans as well.

You can alternate using your tongue and fingers to stimulate her clitoris and just like what's advised above, if she indicates something that's really turning her on, just keep doing it! This is one way on how to make her scream with pleasure.

STEP 4

If clitoral stimulation has not brought on an orgasm yet, then try G-spot stimulation! Assuming that she's already hot and wet, slowly insert your index and middle finger inside her womanhood, palm up. Once inside, position your fingers to the "11 o'clock." Slowly try and locate a small bump or swelling (like an engorged clitoris). Once you find this spot, congratulations... you've located the elusive G-spot!

STEP 5

You can stimulate the G-spot in many ways. You can tap it with your fingers, draw lazy or frenzied circles around it, or flick it wildly like a light switch. If you wish, you can use your thumb to stimulate her clitoris while stimulating her G-spot. This will surely give her an orgasm to be remembered!

CONCLUSION

Here Are Some Key Concepts You Should Keep In Mind:

There are a lot of different little things that you can do to be seen as more attractive through a woman's eyes. Not all of these things have to do with you being rich and handsome. Many of them are easily in your own control.

You can learn how to get the girls to chase you. All it takes is a bit of planning, practice, and effort, so give it a try. Once you figure out the art to being picked up, you will never want to go back to the old way again.

- **Think Like A Woman**. This is hard of course, but the idea is to start slowing things down. Women are really clever and sensitive and they sure know what men want. Be smart. Do not ask her to go to bed with you on your first date. By slowing down the process of seducing a woman, you are already ahead of most of your competitors.

- **Make Plans**. Women love men who know how to plan things. In order to seduce a woman, you must have some sort of plan. Send her an invitation for a dinner you or someone else will prepare. Send her a romantic email (not sexual but romantic and sweet). Leave an envelope with a mysterious and meaningful message on her doorstep. Make sure she knows that you are working hard to seduce her. They just love men who keep trying and make plans to seduce them.

- **Your Appearance:** You don't have to be naturally good looking. There are in fact some disadvantages to being really good looking. One disadvantage is that many women may assume that you are a player. However, you shouldn't let that stop you from improving your appearance.

   What you should do is look at how you dress, your fitness level, your hair, and your body language. The idea is to improve yourself in these areas so that you do look your best. This can help you feel more confident about yourself, and it helps to leave a more positive first impression.

- **The Right Kind Of Compliments:** How you compliment a woman is a big deal if she is the kind of woman who gets them all the time. This is either because she takes those compliments for granted or because she doesn't believe half the things men say to her. So what do you do?

You always compliment a woman on the things that make her unique. Sometimes it just helps to ask yourself why. "You look beautiful" Why does she look so beautiful? She looks beautiful because of that hot skirt she has on. What you do then is compliment her on her skirt. "I love that hot red skirt your wearing. It really makes you stand out from the rest of the girls."

- **Buy Her A Gift**. All women are seduced by gifts even if they don't let it show. You don't have to buy an expensive gift. Buy her a book, a chocolate or something like that. You get the point. A good idea would be to buy her a book with sweet and romantic quotes. Show her that she comes first. This is a great way to seduce a woman.

- **Start Talking**. Make her laugh. Women just love to laugh, it's a fact. They are seduced by men with a quality sense of humor. But do not overdo it. Don't talk too much about yourself or your accomplishments. Don't be selfish. Open your mind. You are not the only man in the world. This is critical. Stay focused on her thoughts and actions. Learn from her.

- **Never Look At Other Women When You Are With Her.** Women hate to be compared to the girl you're looking at. It is men's nature to be looking at women, especially beautiful women. Men will do this until the day they die, but women will never understand this nature. This is due to the biological drive for monogamy in women. The ogling must be minimized when she's around.

- **If You Manage To Touch Her Don't Go For Her Pants Straight Away**. Be sensual and passionate. Most women love to be touched in various places like their necks and shoulders.
  Again, slow down the process. Make them wonder why you are so different from all other guys who just want to get them to take their clothes off. Resist the temptation!

- **Seek common interests**. Common interests or hobbies make relationships last longer. If you have to develop an appreciation for romantic films or foreign languages just to share something in common with her, that's a price worth paying. This is proof that you care about her.

- **You Want To Know More On How To Seduce A Woman**. I know. So stick to the good old "Ladies First." This applies everywhere, but especially in the bedroom. Try your best to please her first. If you are stuck, ask her what would please her. If you give her the ultimate pleasure first you are a winner. You got her. She will beg you for more. And then she will do her best to give you pleasure. And we all know what that means.

There is one important quality that I left out of the mix. That one quality is confidence. Everything that you say to her, and how you behave around her have to indicate that you are comfortable with yourself. All of those other things put together will be meaningless if you can't get that part right. Nevertheless, all of things listed in this book will help you in seducing a woman.

Printed in the USA
CPSIA information can be obtained
at www.ICGtesting.com
LVHW020432220823
755830LV00003BA/303